Healthy living demystified:

A comprehensive guide to simplifying wellness

By

Mary M Bennett

Table of content

Introduction:

Welcome to "Healthy Living Demystified," where we disentangle the intricacies of well-being to make sound residing open and reachable for everybody. In this book, we'll investigate pragmatic techniques, proof-based exhortation, and noteworthy stages to improve on your excursion towards enduring well-being and essentialness. Whether you're a novice or a carefully prepared health lover, this guide will enable you to settle on informed decisions, develop supportable propensities, and flourish as a main priority, body, and soul.

Chapter 1:

Grasping the Underpinnings of Wellbeing

In this primary part, we dive into the center standards of well-being and health. From the significance of sustenance and active work to the job of rest and stress the board, we'll investigate how every part of our way of life adds to generally speaking prosperity. By understanding these essentials, you'll be furnished with the information to establish a strong starting point for your well-being process.

Understanding the groundwork of well-being is principal for keeping up with general prosperity. It incorporates different perspectives, including physical, mental, close-to-home, and social aspects.

First and foremost, actual well-being spins around keeping a fair eating routine, customary activity, sufficient rest, and staying away from destructive substances like tobacco and exorbitant liquor. It's fundamental to pay attention to your body, address any well-being concerns quickly, and participate in preventive medical services measures, for example, immunizations and ordinary check-ups.

Psychological wellness is similarly critical, including close-to-home versatility, stress the executives, and looking for help when required. Rehearsing care, reflection, or participating in leisure activities can advance mental prosperity. Moreover, cultivating sound connections and relational abilities adds to close-to-home strength.

Social well-being stresses the significance of supporting associations with others, cultivating a feeling of having a place, and partaking in friendly exercises. Solid social encouraging groups of people give close-to-home support during testing times and upgrade generally personal satisfaction.

Besides, ecological variables assume a huge part in well-being. Admittance to clean air, water, and safe everyday environments is major for prosperity. Supportable way-of-life decisions, like lessening waste and monitoring normal assets, add to a better planet and, thus, human well-being.

Social and financial factors additionally impact well-being results. Perceiving and tending to aberrations in medical care access and results is pivotal for advancing well-being value and guaranteeing that everybody has the chance to accomplish ideal well-being.

In outline, understanding the groundwork of well-being includes tending to physical, mental, profound, social, ecological, social, and financial variables. By adopting a comprehensive strategy and settling on educated decisions regarding these regions, people can endeavour to accomplish and keep up with ideal well-being and prosperity.

Chapter 2:

Dominating Sustenance Nuts and bolts

Sustenance doesn't need to be muddled. Here, we work on the study of eating great by zeroing in on entire, supplement-thick food sources. You'll figure out how to explore the supermarket with certainty, interpret food marks, and make adjusted dinners that support your body and fulfill your taste buds. Express farewell to prohibitive weight control plans and hi a reasonable way to deal with eating for wellbeing and satisfaction.

Dominating sustenance rudiments is fundamental for keeping up with ideal well-being and prosperity. It includes grasping the job of supplements, going with informed food decisions, and taking on good dieting propensities.

1. Understanding Macronutrients: Macronutrients are the principal parts of our eating regimen and

incorporate starches, proteins, and fats. Starches give energy, proteins are fundamental for building and fixing tissues, and fats assume a part in cell capability and supplement retention.

2. Balanced Eating regimen: A reasonable eating routine comprises of various food varieties from all nutritional categories. This consist of organic products, vegetables, entire grains, lean proteins, and sound fats. Take a stab at assortment, balance, and piece control to guarantee you get every one of the fundamental supplements your body needs.

3. Micronutrients: notwithstanding macronutrients, micronutrients, for example, nutrients and minerals are essential for by and large wellbeing. Eating a different scope of food varieties guarantees you get a sufficient admission of micronutrients. Consider consolidating supplement-thick food sources like salad greens, nuts, seeds, and vegetables into your eating routine.

4. Hydration: Remaining hydrated is fundamental for different physical processes, including temperature guidelines, absorption, and supplement transport. Intend to drink a lot of water throughout

the day and break point utilization of sweet refreshments.

5. Mindful Eating: Practice careful eating by focusing on craving and totality signals, as well as the taste, surface, and delight in food. Stay away from interruptions while eating, like sitting in front of the television or looking at your telephone, to advance better processing and fulfillment.

6. Portion Control: Be aware of piece sizes to forestall gorging. Utilise obvious prompts, for example, contrasting part estimates with regular articles or utilising more modest plates, to assist with controlling piece sizes.

7. Reading Food Marks: Figure out how to peruse food names to go with informed decisions about the items you devour. Focus on serving sizes, fixing records, and wholesome data, including calories, macronutrients, and micronutrients.

8. Meal Preparation and Arrangement: Plan and get ready for feasts early on to guarantee you have nutritious choices promptly accessible. This can

assist with forestalling hasty food decisions and setting aside time and cash over the long haul.

9. Healthy Eating Examples: Embracing good dieting designs, like the Mediterranean eating routine or Run (Dietary Ways to deal with Stop Hypertension) diet, can give direction on integrating nutritious food sources into your everyday practice.

10. Seeking Expert Direction: If you have explicit dietary requirements or well-being concerns, consider counselling an enrolled dietitian or nutritionist for customised direction and backing.

By dominating sustenance nuts and bolts and embracing good dieting propensities, you can uphold your general well-being and prosperity for quite a long time into the future. Recollect that little, maintainable changes can prompt critical enhancements in your well-being over the long run.

Chapter 3:

Moving Your Body with Delight

Exercise ought to be a wellspring of euphoria, not an errand.

Here, we investigate various proactive tasks that take care of various interests, capacities, and inclinations. From lively strolls in nature to extreme cardio exercise, you'll find endless ways of moving your body and receive the rewards of standard activity. We'll likewise talk about procedures for beating normal boundaries to actual work and remaining inspired for the long stretch.

Moving your body with bliss is a brilliant method for focusing on your physical and mental prosperity while embracing a positive relationship with exercise and development. Here is an extensive aide on the most proficient method to imbue delight into your actual work schedule:

1. Find Exercises You Love: Investigate different types of actual work, like moving, climbing, swimming, yoga, or cycling, to find what gives you pleasure. Pick exercises that impact you and cause you to feel eager to move your body.

2. Embrace Perkiness: Move toward practice with a fun-loving mentality. Permit yourself to be unconstrained, explore different avenues regarding various developments, and let go of self-judgment. Recollect that moving your body ought to be fun and charming.

3. Set Sensible Objectives: Put forth practical and reachable objectives that line up with your inclinations and capacities. Rather than zeroing in exclusively on results like weight reduction or muscle gain, focus on objectives connected with how development affects you and the delight it brings into your life.

4. Listen to Your Body: Focus on how your body feels during actual work. Honor your body's prompts and limits, and change your exercise power or span on a case-by-case basis. Recall that rest and

recuperation are fundamental parts of a decent wellness schedule.

5. Connect with Nature: Exploit outside exercises to associate with nature while moving your body. Whether it's going for a climb in the mountains, a stroll on the oceanfront, or rehearsing yoga in the recreation area, investing energy outside can upgrade your feeling of prosperity and satisfaction.

6. Cultivate Care: Practice care during active work by being completely present at the time. Center around the vibes of development, the mood of your breath, and the magnificence of your environmental factors. Careful development can extend your association with your body and enhance sensations of happiness.

7. Invite Social Association: Offer your delight of development with others by practicing with companions, and relatives, or joining a bunch of wellness classes or sports groups. Building a steady local area around actual work can improve inspiration and pleasure.

8. Celebrate Advancement: Commend your advancement and accomplishments along your wellness process, regardless of how little. Recognize the work you put into moving your body and the positive effect it has on your general prosperity.

9. Mix It Up: Keep your workout routine new and energizing by integrating assortment into your exercises. Attempt new exercises, change around your routine consistently, and challenge yourself to step beyond your usual range of familiarity.

10. Practice Appreciation: Develop an appreciation for your body's capacity to move and for the delight that actual work brings into your life. Express appreciation for the potential chance to participate in development, no matter what your wellness level or capacities.

By moving your body with satisfaction and integrating these standards into your wellness schedule, you can encourage a positive relationship with work out, improve your general prosperity, and develop a deep-rooted obligation to remain dynamic and sound. Recall that bliss is a strong inspiration, so focus on exercises that give you joy and satisfaction.

Chapter 4:

Developing Mental Prosperity

Genuine well-being envelops something other than actual well-being — it's likewise about sustaining our psychological and profound prosperity. Here, we investigate care rehearses, stress-decrease procedures, and systems for cultivating strength notwithstanding life's difficulties. By focusing on taking care of oneself and self-empathy, you'll develop a positive outlook and inward harmony that emanates outward into each part of your life.

Developing mental prosperity is a deep-rooted venture that includes supporting your profound, mental, and social well-being. Here is an extensive aide on the most proficient method to encourage mental prosperity:

1. Self-Mindfulness: Start by developing mindfulness and figuring out your viewpoints, sentiments, and ways of behaving. Practice care procedures like reflection, profound breathing, or

journaling to notice your internal encounters without judgment.

2. Emotional Guideline: Learn sound ways of adapting to and controlling your feelings. Foster systems like profound breathing activities, moderate muscle unwinding, or taking part in imaginative outlets like workmanship or music to oversee pressure and tension.

3. Positive Connections: Develop steady and significant associations with companions, family, and local area individuals. Put time and exertion into sustaining these associations, as friendly help is fundamental for keeping up with mental prosperity.

4. Boundaries: Lay out solid limits to safeguard your psychological and profound well-being. Figure out how to decisively convey your necessities and cutoff points, and focus on taking care of yourself with exercises that re-energize and revive you.

5. Healthy Way of Life Propensities: Take on propensities that help your general prosperity, including standard activity, adjusted nourishment, satisfactory rest, and staying away from hurtful

substances like medications and liquor. Actual well-being and psychological well-being are firmly interconnected.

6. Mindful Utilization: Be aware of what you consume, including media, news, and online entertainment. Limit openness to negative or troubling substances, and search out wellsprings of motivation, energy, and chuckling.

7. Meaningful Exercises: Take part in exercises that give you pleasure, satisfaction, and a feeling of direction. Whether it's seeking after-leisure activities, chipping in, or investing energy in nature, focus on exercises that support your spirit and touch off your enthusiasm.

8. Seeking Help: Connect for proficient assistance assuming you're battling with your psychological well-being. Treatment, advising, or upholding gatherings can give important assets and direction to exploring difficulties and building strength.

9. Gratitude Practice: Develop a mentality of appreciation by routinely communicating appreciation for individuals, encounters, and favors

in your day-to-day existence. Rehearsing appreciation can move your viewpoint and increment sensations of bliss and happiness.

10. Continuous Development: Embrace a development outlook and view difficulties as any open doors for learning and self-awareness. Develop versatility by adjusting to misfortune and returning from difficulties with flexibility and hopefulness.

11. Savouring Minutes: Set aside some margin to enjoy and value the current second. Carefully participate in exercises, appreciating the sights, sounds, and sensations around you. By dialling back and being completely present, you can develop a more noteworthy feeling of harmony and satisfaction.

12. Self-Sympathy: Be thoughtful and humane toward yourself, particularly during seasons of battle or trouble. Practice self-sympathy by treating yourself with similar warmth and understanding you would propose to a dear companion.

By integrating these practices into your routine, you can develop mental prosperity, assemble versatility, and flourish in all aspects of your life. Recollect that emotional wellness is an excursion, and looking for help and direction en route is OK. Focus on your psychological prosperity, and recollect that you have the right to carry on with a satisfying and significant life

Chapter 5:

Making Solid Propensities that Stick

In this part, we jump into the study of conduct change and propensity development. You'll figure out how to lay out sensible objectives, make successful activity plans, and remain responsible to yourself en route. Whether you're hoping to lay out a reliable workout daily schedule, further develop your dietary patterns, or focus on rest, you'll find pragmatic procedures for building sound propensities that endure for an extremely long period.

Making sound propensities that stick includes understanding the brain science behind propensity development and carrying out systems to help long-haul conduct change. Here is an itemized note on the cycle:

Figuring out Propensity Arrangement:

1. Cue: This is the trigger that starts the way of behaving. It tends to be day, a particular spot, a close-to-home state, or a former activity.

2. Routine: The actual conduct. This can be anything from practicing to having a serving of mixed greens for lunch.

3. Reward: The uplifting feedback that follows the way of behaving, which builds up the propensity circle. It very well may be physical (like the arrival of endorphins in the wake of working out) or mental (feeling refined or assuaged).

Methodologies for Making Sound Propensities:

1. Start Little: Start with minuscule, reasonable changes instead of overpowering yourself with uncommon movements. For instance, if you need to begin working out, focus on only five minutes daily at first.

2. Set Clear Objectives: Characterise explicit, quantifiable, attainable, pertinent, and time-bound (Shrewd) objectives. This clearness assists you with keeping on track and keeping tabs on your development.

3. Use Execution Expectations: Plan out when and where you will play out your new propensity. This

improves the probability of finishing by lessening choice exhaustion and depending on autopilot.

4. Create Responsibility: Offer your objectives with a companion, join a care group, or recruit a mentor. Being responsible to another person can assist you with remaining committed when inspiration winds down.

5. Track Your Advancement: Keep a diary or use propensity following applications to screen your way of behaving and celebrate little wins en route.

6. Stay Adaptable: Be available to change your methodology if something isn't working. Variation is vital to supporting propensities over the long haul.

7. Focus on Consistency, Not Flawlessness: Go for the gold flawlessness. Reliably rehearsing a way of behaving, even defectively, is more helpful than irregular explosions of exertion.

8. Practice Self-Sympathy: Be caring to yourself when you experience mishaps. Rather than criticising yourself, use difficulties as learning amazing open doors and commit once again to your objectives.

9. Create a Strong Climate: Encircle yourself with individuals who urge and rouse you to keep up with your sound propensities. Also, eliminate or limit sets

that might entice you to return to old, unfortunate ways of behaving.

10. Celebrate Achievements: Recognize and remunerate yourself for arriving at achievements en route. Indulge yourself with something uniquely amazing or participate in exercises that give you pleasure.

Keeping up with Solid Propensities:

1. Stay Careful: Ceaselessly help yourself to remember the advantages of your new propensities and the motivations behind why you began.

2. Review and Change: Routinely assess your headway and make changes on a case-by-case basis to guarantee your propensities stay lined up with your objectives and way of life.

3. Plan for Hindrances: Expect difficulties that might emerge and foster techniques to conquer them. This proactive methodology will assist you with exploring misfortunes all the more successfully.

4. Practice Appreciation: Develop a feeling of appreciation for the chance to focus on your well-being and prosperity through your propensities. This positive outlook can fuel your inspiration and strength.

By carrying out these methodologies and understanding the brain research of propensity development, you can make solid propensities that become a necessary piece of your way of life, prompting durable positive change.

Chapter 6:

Exploring Social and Natural Impacts

Our social and natural environmental elements assume a huge part in forming our well-being and ways of behaving. In this section, we'll investigate how to explore peer pressure, normal practices, and outside impacts that might affect your health process. From defining limits to looking for help from similar people, you'll figure out how to establish a strong climate that enables you to flourish.

Exploring social and natural impacts is fundamental for keeping up with prosperity and settling on informed choices that line up with your qualities and objectives. Here is an exhaustive aide on the most proficient method to explore these impacts really:

1. Awareness: Begin by developing familiarity with the social and ecological variables that influence your life. This incorporates perceiving the standards, assumptions, and tensions inside your groups of friends, as well as figuring out the ecological variables that influence your day-to-day decisions and ways of behaving.

2. Critical Reasoning: Foster decisive reasoning abilities to assess the data and messages you get from social and natural sources. Question presumptions, think about alternate points of view, and search out dependable wellsprings of data to go with informed choices.

3. Personal Qualities: Explain your qualities and needs to direct your dynamic cycle. Consider what makes the biggest difference to you throughout everyday life, whether it's well-being, supportability, civil rights, or different standards, and utilize these qualities as a compass to explore social and natural impacts.

4. Boundaries: Lay out sound limits to safeguard your prosperity and keep up with independence in your decisions. Figure out how to express no to

prevailing burdens or natural impacts that contention with your qualities or objectives, and focus on exercises and connections that line up with your needs.

5. Peer Impact: Be aware of the impact of friends and gatherings on your way of behaving and independent direction. Encircle yourself with steady and positive impacts who regard your qualities and energize your development and prosperity.

6. Media Education: Foster media proficiency abilities to fundamentally assess the data and messages depicted in news sources, including online entertainment, news, and promotion. Knowing about the substance you consume and thinking about its likely effect on your perspectives and ways of behaving.

7. Advocacy: Backer for social and natural causes that line up with your qualities and convictions. Engage in local area drives, humanitarian efforts, or backing efforts to have a constructive outcome in your general surroundings.

8. Adaptability: Develop flexibility and strength to explore changing social and ecological settings. Perceive that cultural standards and natural circumstances might advance over the long haul, and be available to change your convictions and ways of behaving likewise.

9. Sustainability Practices: Integrate maintainable practices into your day-to-day routine to limit your natural effect and advance a better planet. This might incorporate decreasing waste, preserving energy and water, supporting eco-accommodating organizations, and pushing for natural arrangements.

10. Community Commitment: Draw in with your local area to encourage social associations, support neighbourhood drives, and address social issues cooperatively. Building solid local area ties can give a feeling of having a place and strengthening in exploring social and natural impacts.

11. Continuous Learning: Remain educated and taught about friendly and natural issues through continuous learning and exchange. Go to studios, workshops, or local area occasions, and take part in

discussions with others to develop your comprehension and viewpoint.

By exploring social and ecological impacts with mindfulness, decisive reasoning, and arrangement with your qualities, you can engage yourself to settle on decisions that advance prosperity for you and others, while adding to positive social and natural change. Recall that your activities can make expanding influences that stretch out a long way past yourself, molding the world for people in the future.

Chapter 7:

Embracing a Decent Way of Life

Balance is the way to manageable health. In this section, we'll talk about the significance of tracking down amicability in all aspects of your life, from work and connections to recreation and taking care of oneself. You'll figure out how to focus on your significant investment, put down stopping points, and practice taking care of yourself without responsibility or burnout.

By embracing balance, you'll make a day-to-day existence that feeds your body, brain, and soul.

Embracing a fair way of life is fundamental for advancing in general prosperity and satisfaction in all everyday issues. It includes incorporating different aspects, including actual well-being, mental and profound prosperity, connections, work, relaxation, and self-awareness, to make concordance and fulfillment. Here is an exhaustive aide on the most proficient method to embrace a decent way of life:

1. Prioritize Taking care of oneself: Make taking care of oneself a non-debatable piece of your daily practice. This incorporates dealing with your actual well-being through ordinary activity, adjusted nourishment, satisfactory rest, and preventive medical care rehearses. Also, focus on exercises that feed your psychological and close-to-home prosperity, like care, unwinding strategies, and side interests that give you pleasure.

2. Set Limits: Lay out sound limits to safeguard your time, energy, and needs. Figure out how to express no to exercises or responsibilities that overpower or deplete you, and focus on exercises that line up with your qualities and objectives. Defining limits permits you to zero in on the main thing and forestalls burnout.

3. Manage Pressure: Foster powerful pressure on the executive's methods to adapt to life's difficulties and vulnerabilities. This might incorporate care

reflection, profound breathing activities, yoga, journaling, or looking for help from companions, family, or emotional wellness experts. By overseeing pressure, you can improve versatility and keep a feeling of equilibrium amid misfortune.

4. Cultivate Significant Connections: Put time and exertion into sustaining strong and significant associations with companions, family, and local area individuals. Focus on quality time enjoyed with friends and family, take part in transparent correspondence, and proposition backing and support to other people. Significant associations give a feeling of having a place and backing during both upbeat and troublesome times.

5. Work-Life Equilibrium: Endeavor to accomplish a good overall arrangement between work and individual life. Put down stopping points around work hours, enjoy ordinary reprieves, and set aside a few minutes for recreation exercises, side interests, and associating beyond work. Recall that focusing on taking care of oneself and individual time eventually improves efficiency, innovativeness, and occupation fulfillment.

6. Continuous Learning and Development: Cultivate a development outlook by embracing valuable open doors for learning and self-improvement. Search out new difficulties, seek after interests and interests, and participate in deep-rooted learning through courses, studios, or self-study. Embracing development and advancement improves educational encounters and upgrades general satisfaction.

7. Practice Appreciation: Develop a demeanor of appreciation by routinely communicating appreciation for individuals, encounters, and favors in your day-to-day existence. Keep an appreciation diary, ponder positive minutes, and offer thanks to others through thoughtful gestures and appreciation. Appreciation cultivates inspiration, flexibility, and a more profound appreciation for life's gifts.

8. Live with Expectation: Live with aim and reason by adjusting your activities to your qualities, objectives, and goals. Put forth significant objectives that move and rouse you, and make purposeful strides towards accomplishing them. By living purposefully, you gain an ability to know east from west and satisfaction in your life.

9. Embrace Adaptability: Be available to adjust and change your arrangements depending on the situation in light of changing conditions or needs. Embracing adaptability permits you to stream with life's high points and low points, explore difficulties with versatility, and take full advantage of chances as they emerge.

10. Nourish Your Spirit: At last, focus on exercises that feed your spirit and give you a feeling of pleasure, reason, and satisfaction. Whether it's investing energy in nature, seeking after imaginative undertakings, chipping in, or rehearsing thoughtful gestures, set aside a few minutes for exercises that elevate and motivate you.

By embracing a fair way of life that focuses on taking care of oneself, significant connections, self-awareness, and living with expectations, you can develop more prominent joy, satisfaction, and prosperity in all parts of your life. Recollect that equilibrium is a powerful cycle that requires continuous consideration and change, so be thoughtful and patient with yourself as you explore the excursion toward all-encompassing prosperity.

Chapter 8:

Conquering Difficulties and Remaining Tough

No well-being venture is without its difficulties. In this part, we'll investigate normal impediments that might emerge en route, from mishaps and levels to self-uncertainty and negative self-talk. You'll figure out how to develop versatility, flexibility, and self-sympathy to defeat hindrances and remain focused on your objectives. With the right attitude and emotionally supportive network, you'll become more grounded and stronger than at any other time.

Beating difficulties and remaining strong is a basic part of self-improvement and exploring life's promising and less promising times with elegance and strength. Strength is the capacity to adjust and return from affliction, misfortunes, and stressors, and it very well may be developed through different procedures and practices.

Here is a complete aide on the most proficient method to defeat difficulties and remain versatile:

1. Develop a Development Mentality: Develop a development outlook, which is the conviction that difficulties and misfortunes are potential open doors for learning and development instead of inconceivable snags. Embrace disappointments and mishaps as significant opportunities for growth that can eventually reinforce your flexibility and character.

2. Build Mindfulness: Foster mindfulness to perceive your assets, shortcomings, and methods for dealing with hardship or stress. Comprehend how you ordinarily answer difficulties and stressors and distinguish regions for development and improvement. Mindfulness permits you to pursue cognizant decisions and answer actually to affliction.

3. Foster Social Help: Develop serious areas of strength for an organization of companions, family,

tutors, and local area individuals who can offer consolation, direction, and basic reassurance during troublesome times. Connect with confided-in people when you want help or a listening ear, and respond with support when others are confronting difficulties.

4. Practice Versatility: Foster flexibility and adaptability to explore changing conditions and startling difficulties. Embrace vulnerability as a characteristic piece of life, and spotlight on finding intelligent fixes and options when confronted with impediments. Flexibility permits you to flourish in powerful and flighty conditions.

5. Cultivate Survival techniques: Construct a tool kit of sound methods for dealing with especially difficult times to oversee pressure, nervousness, and misfortune. This might incorporate care reflection, profound breathing activities, actual work, journaling, innovative articulation, or looking for proficient help from specialists or advisors. Try different things with various methods to find what turns out best for you.

6. Maintain Point of view: Keep a fair point of view and stay away from catastrophizing or amplifying difficulties messed up. Perceive that misfortunes and hardships are transitory and that you have the strength and versatility to beat them. Centre around the current second and what you have some control over, as opposed to harping on remorseful thoughts or agonising over what's to come.

7. Set Reasonable Objectives: Put forth practical and feasible objectives that give guidance and inspiration during testing times. Break bigger objectives into more modest, sensible advances, and praise progress and achievements en route. Putting forth objectives keeps up with concentration and energy, in any event, when confronted with obstructions.

8. Practice Self-Empathy: Be thoughtful and empathetic toward yourself, particularly during seasons of battle or disappointment. Indulge yourself with a similar sympathy and understanding you would propose to a dear companion, and stay away from self-analysis or unforgiving judgment. Self-sympathy cultivates versatility and reinforces your capacity to return from misfortunes.

9. Seek Significance and Reason: Track down the importance and reason in your encounters, even despite the difficulty. Interface with your qualities, interests, and feelings of direction, and draw upon them as wellsprings of inspiration and strength. Develop an appreciation for the illustrations learned and the amazing open doors for development that difficulties give.

10. Embrace Learning experiences: Embrace difficulties as any open doors for self-awareness, self-revelation, and change. View mishaps as diversions as opposed to impasses, and confidence in your capacity to explore the excursion toward flexibility and prosperity. Recall that flexibility isn't tied in with staying away from difficulties but rather turning around them with boldness, strength, and assurance.

By integrating these systems into your life, you can defeat difficulties and afflictions with flexibility and effortlessness, becoming more grounded, smarter, and more engaged than previously. Recall that versatility is an expertise that can be developed and reinforced over the long haul and that each challenge you face is a potential chance to develop and flourish.

Chapter 9:

Observing Your Triumphs

In this part, we commend your excursion towards further developed well-being and prosperity. You'll think about your accomplishments, of all shapes and sizes, and recognize the headway you've made en route. Whether you've arrived at an achievement, defeated a test, or just remained focused on your objectives, it's vital to commend your victories and recognize the difficult work and devotion that got you there.

Commending your victories is a significant part of keeping up with inspiration, supporting confidence, and cultivating a positive mentality. It permits you to recognize your accomplishments, regardless of how large or little, and builds up your feeling of progress and achievement. Here is an exhaustive aide on the most proficient method to praise your triumphs:

1. Acknowledge Your Accomplishments: Carve out the opportunity to recognize and perceive your achievements, regardless of how unassuming they might appear. Whether you've accomplished a significant achievement or followed through with a little responsibility, give yourself credit for your endeavours and the headway you've made.

2. Reflect on Your Excursion: Consider the excursion that prompted your prosperity and value the difficult work, commitment, and steadiness it required. Perceive the obstructions you survived, the examples you learned, and the development you encountered en route. Praise the versatility and assurance that pushed you forward.

3. Celebrate Achievements: Separate your bigger objectives into more modest achievements and praise them at all times. Whether it's arriving at a specific cutoff time, meeting a business target, or dominating another expertise, carve out

opportunities to praise your advancement and achievements. Praising achievements keeps you roused and propelled to push ahead.

4. Share Your Triumphs: Offer your victories to others, whether it's companions, family, partners, or coaches. Praise your accomplishments transparently and energetically, and permit others to partake in your satisfaction and fervour. Sharing your victories builds up your feeling of achievement as well as rouses and persuades others to seek after their objectives.

5. Reward Yourself: Indulge yourself with a prize or guilty pleasure as an approach to praising your victories. Whether it's a unique dinner, a loosening up spa day, or a little extravagance thing you've been looking at, pick a prize that feels significant and compensating to you. Remunerating yourself supports a positive way of behaving and energizes you to proceed with progress.

6. Express Appreciation: Offer thanks for the help, support, and open doors that added to your prosperity. Thank the people who have upheld and trusted you en route, whether it's companions,

family, tutors, or partners. Appreciation develops a feeling of association and appreciation for the connections and assets that have assisted you with succeeding.

7. Document Your Accomplishments: Track your victories and accomplishments as an approach to praising your advancement and building fearlessness. Whether it's a diary, a dream board, or a computerised portfolio, report your achievements and return to them consistently to help yourself remember how far you've come.

8. Set New Objectives: Utilise your triumphs as energy to lay out new objectives and goals for what's in store. Expand on your accomplishments by provoking yourself to arrive at new levels and seek after new open doors. Defining new objectives keeps you engaged, propelled, and taking part in proceeding with development and advancement.

9. Practice Self-Sympathy: Be caring and sympathetic toward yourself, particularly assuming you experience mishaps or difficulties en route. Praise your victories with confidence and appreciation, and perceive that misfortunes are a

characteristic piece of the excursion toward progress. Indulge yourself with a similar benevolence and understanding you would propose to a companion.

10. Celebrate Your Exceptional Excursion: Praise your achievements in a novel manner that feels bona fide and significant to you. Whether you lean toward a calm reflection, a vivacious social occasion with friends and family, or an individual custom of appreciation, celebrate such that respects your singularity and mirrors your qualities and inclinations.

By commending your triumphs, you recognize your accomplishments as well as develop a positive outlook, fabricate self-assurance, and move forward with development and outcome later on. Make sure to commend yourself frequently and embrace the excursion of self-disclosure and accomplishment with satisfaction and appreciation.

Chapter 10:

Supporting Your Sound Way of Life forever

At last, we'll talk about methodologies for keeping up with your recently discovered well-being and health as long as possible. You'll figure out how to incorporate solid propensities into your everyday daily schedule, adjust to life's inescapable changes, and keep advancing on your health process. By focusing on deep-rooted learning, development, and self-disclosure, you'll make an energetic and satisfying life that mirrors your qualities and needs.

Supporting a sound way of life for life is tied in with making long-haul, economic changes that help your physical, mental, and close-to-home prosperity. It includes embracing sound propensities, focusing on taking care of oneself, and developing a positive mentality that permits you to explore life's difficulties with versatility and elegance. Here is a complete aide on the most proficient method to support your sound way of life forever:

1. Focus on Equilibrium: Embrace a fair way to deal with well-being that incorporates sustaining your body with nutritious food varieties, remaining dynamic, getting sufficient rest, overseeing pressure, and focusing on taking care of oneself. Stay away from outrageous weight control plans or exercise regimens that are not reasonable over the long haul.

2. Set Sensible Objectives: Put forth reasonable and attainable objectives that line up with your qualities, needs, and way of life. Break bigger objectives into more modest, sensible advances, and commend your advancement en route. Putting forth feasible objectives keeps up with inspiration and forestall burnout.

3. Find Exercises You Appreciate: Take part in proactive tasks and activities that you appreciate and anticipate. Whether it's moving, climbing, swimming, yoga, or group activities, pick exercises

that give you pleasure and satisfaction. Partaking in your exercises makes it simpler to remain reliable and keep a functioning way of life.

4. Create Solid Propensities: Lay out sound propensities that become imbued in your day-to-day daily schedule. This might incorporate feast preparation, planning customary activity meetings, rehearsing care or contemplation, and focusing on sufficient rest. Consistency is vital to supporting a solid way of life after some time.

5. Practise Careful Eating: Foster a careful way to deal with eating by focusing on craving and completion signs, relishing each chomp, and picking food varieties that feed your body and fulfil your taste buds. Keep away from prohibitive weight control plans and on second thought centre around making adjusted, nutritious decisions that help your general prosperity.

6. Build an Emotionally supportive network: Encircle yourself with a strong organisation of companions, family, and similar people who urge and rouse you to focus on your well-being. Share your objectives, difficulties, and victories with

others, and rest on your emotionally supportive network for responsibility and inspiration.

7. Be Adaptable and Versatile: Be adaptable and versatile in your way of dealing with well-being and health. Life is brimming with startling exciting bends in the road, so be ready to change your schedules and plans depending on the situation. Embrace change with a receptive outlook and view difficulties as any open doors for development and learning.

8. Practice Self-Sympathy: Be thoughtful and empathetic toward yourself, particularly when you experience mishaps or difficulties en route. Indulge yourself with a similar sympathy and understanding you would propose to a companion, and stay away from self-analysis or negative self-talk. Recollect that progress isn't generally straight, and each forward-moving step is a triumph worth celebrating.

9. Celebrate Your Advancement: Commend your advancement and achievements, regardless of how little. Carve out the opportunity to recognize and value the positive changes you've made in your life, and perceive the work and devotion it took to arrive.

Commending your victories builds up your obligation to keep a sound way of life forever.

10. Stay Taught and Informed: Remain instructed and informed about well-being and health subjects, however, be knowing of the data you consume. Search out trustworthy wellsprings of data and talk with medical care experts or enlisted dietitians assuming that you have different kinds of feedback. Remain open to new research and advancements in the field of well-being and health, and change your propensities and practices likewise.

By integrating these methodologies into your life, you can support a solid way of life forever and partake in the advantages of working on actual well-being, mental prosperity, and general personal satisfaction. Recall that keeping a sound way of life is a continuous excursion, so show restraint toward yourself and commend your advancement constantly.

Conclusion:

Congrats on finishing "Healthy Living Demystified"! Outfitted with the information, abilities, and certainty acquired from this book, you're exceptional to leave on an excursion towards enduring well-being and imperativeness. Keep in mind that wellbeing is a long-lasting pursuit, and each step you steer towards better wellbeing is a positive development. Here's to your proceeding with progress and prosperity!

www.ingramcontent.com/pod-product-compliance
Lightning Source LLC
Chambersburg PA
CBHW070733260726
48660CB00007B/2825